WRITING THE NURSING RESUME

Little Twin Stars

Lourdes Fabricio
2876 20th St.
San Pablo, CA 94806

©1976.1988 SANRIO CO.,LTD.

TABLE OF CONTENTS

	PAGE
OVERVIEW	1
The Importance of a Good Resume	3
Nurse Recruiters Answer Your Questions	4
Nine Steps for Developing A Professional Resume	8
STEP 1 – CHOOSE A FORMAT	9
Chronological Resume	10
Functional Resume	12
Combination Resume	14
STEP 2 – PLAN THE CONTENT	18
STEP 3 – TAKE AN INVENTORY OF YOUR SKILLS	22
Job Inventory Form	23
STEP 4 – DEVELOP SKILL DESCRIPTIONS	27
Word List	30
Action Phrases	31
STEP 5 – WRITE THE FIRST DRAFT	33
First Draft Example	41
STEP 6 – WRITE THE FINAL DRAFT	43
Final Draft Example	49
STEP 7 – PRODUCE YOUR RESUME	51
Chronological Resume	52
Functional Resume	54
Combination Resume	56
STEP 8 – WRITE THE COVER LETTER	58
Example For a Recent BSN Graduate	60

Example For a Nursing Administrator   61

Example For an Unsolicited Inquiry   62

STEP 9 – CHECK YOUR RESUME AND COVER LETTER   63

OVERVIEW

What can a good resume do for you? By itself,
a good resume won't get you a job. However,
it can get you the interview that eventually
leads to a job offer.

The most important thing to remember in seeking
a new position is that your biggest problem is
your competition. Specifically, competition
that is represented by scores of other resumes.
It is not uncommon, for example, for a nursing
recruiter to receive over 300 resumes for one
advertised position.

How can you increase the chances of your resume
being selected from among so many? If you
remember that you face stiff competition, it
becomes apparent that your resume must do
certain things for you. It must:

o   look and sound professional

o   sell your abilities quickly and concisely

In short, your resume must say: "This is the
resume of a candidate who has something valuable
to offer the organization. This is the resume
of a candidate to interview."

On the following pages, you will find outlined
nine steps for preparing a resume. If you follow
these steps carefully, your chances for developing
a professional resume that stands out from the
crowd will be greatly enhanced.

How This Guide is Unique. While there are many
books available on resume writing, this one is
unique in that it:

o   is devoted exclusively to nurses

o   does more than simply tell you how to
    write a resume – it shows you the step-by-
    step process of producing an effective
    resume

o   tells you what nursing recruiters look
    for in a good resume

Who Needs This Guide? This guide is useful for nurses who want to:

o obtain their first entry-level staff position

o obtain higher staff level hospital positions

o move up into hospital management

o return to their careers after a lengthy absence from nursing

o transfer into private business

What are the Objectives of the Guide? This guide will:

o describe what a good resume is and tell you what it can – and cannot – do to help you find the job you want

o give you the three basic resume formats and explain how to choose the one that's best for you

o show you the step-by-step procedure for putting together a winning resume

o tell you how to handle such issues as frequent job changes, changing career directions within nursing, or returning to nursing after a long absence

o explain how to produce a resume that looks professional

o show you how to write an effective cover letter

o give practical answers to the questions most frequently asked by nurses looking for better jobs

THE IMPORTANCE OF A GOOD RESUME

A good resume is very important. It:

- o creates an instantly favorable impression of you

- o immediately relates your avilability to the needs of
    the person who is hiring

- o focuses attention on your special abilities for the specific
    job you want

- o excites interest in you as a potential employee

- o is attractive to the eye and dignified in appearance so that
    it stands a good chance of being selected from among many
    others that may be submitted

- o covers the major strengths you offer and yet is not so long
    that recruiters or potential employers will not want to read it

- o creates the desire to meet you and find out more about you

- o provides a complete document that recruiters or potential
    employers can refer to throughout the hiring process

In addition to helping you seek a job, your resume can assist you in:

- o applying for advanced nursing education opportunities

- o submitting credentials to professional and honor societies

- o submitting your credentials for presentations at profes-
    sional and community programs

- o being nominated for office in professional and/or community
    programs

- o obtaining consultation assignments

- o networking

NURSE RECRUITERS ANSWER YOUR QUESTIONS

We interviewed nursing recruiters at hospitals, clinics, and other health care organizations to find out what they are seeking in job candidates. Here is a report on our findings.

Q: In general, how would you describe today's job market for nurses?

A: Job recruitment is increasingly a "buyers' market." As hospitals lose patient population, they must cut staff. Consequently, hospitals are looking for nurses with experience in specific disciplines. In addition, many nurses have to accept positions on the less desirable second and third work shifts.

The most significant trend we discovered is toward specialization. Many hospitals are in the market for applicants experienced in critical care, primary care, obstetric/gynecologic, ontologic, rehabilitation, and psychiatric nursing. It is important that you focus in on the specialty you want to pursue, acquire the necessary education and certification, and then build your experience in this area.

Q: How is the job market at HMOs and clinics?

A: The market seems more promising for nurses in these organizations. They are looking for the same skills that hospitals are seeking.

Q: How good are the job opportunities for recent graduates?

A: In this tight job market, there is less demand than before for recent graduates with little or no experience. There are two reasons for this. First, there are many experienced nurses looking for jobs. Second, because many hospitals have had to cut staff, they no longer have the programs to give new nurses training and close supervision.

Q: Where should recent graduates apply for positions?

A: The three most promising areas for recent graduates are within large hospital organizations, at clinics, and in some of the newer fields, such as occupational health services. Many of the larger hospitals still have training programs for new nurses. In many instances, these hospitals prefer to hire inexperienced nurses so that they can train them in their procedures. Clinics often will hire and train new graduates because they can be closely supervised by doctors and other nurses. Positions in occupational health services are opening up in businesses that hire nurses to monitor employees who are constantly exposed to chemicals and other potentially dangerous substances. For these positions, the appropriate education and certification is always as important as professional experience.

Q: Are hospitals hiring nurses who are returning to the field after a long absence?

A: In general, the market is difficult for returning nurses. As one recruiter told us: "Because of new medications and technologies, nursing has changed so much over the past few years, it is difficult for returning nurses to be effective." Most institutions require returning nurses to take a five to six month refresher course before they will be considered for a position.

Q: How important are educational credentials in obtaining a position?

A: The specific institution where you received your degree does not appear to be that important. Many facilities prefer diploma nurses over degreed nurses. Other facilities require at least a BSN. For management positions, an advanced degree is often required.

Q: How important is it to show previous job stability?

A: Many hospitals feel that prior job stability is not that important. If you spend an average of $1\frac{1}{2}$ to 2 years in each position, your chances of being hired are very good. However, if you have a record of a few weeks or months at many different hospitals, recruiters will have a less favorable impression.

Q: Are personal and professional references important?

A: The importance of references varies greatly from institution to institution. Many place great emphasis on both professional and personal references. Others simply verify your employment record.

Q: Do hospitals try to promote from within?

A: Virtually every nurse recruiter said their hospital tries to promote from within.

Q: What are nurse recruiters looking for in a resume?

A: Nurse recruiters recommend the following about your resume. It should:

> look professional
>
> be well written, with no grammatical or spelling errors
>
> be concise and to the point
>
> give the relevant information – for example if you were a head nurse, they want to know where, the number of people you supervised, your duties, and your accomplishments
>
> list certification courses and published articles only that are relevant to the position you are seeking

Q: What do nurse recruiters look for in a cover letter?

A: They advise that your letter should :

> be concise and clear about the job you are seeking

> recap your relevant experience

> tell whether you want part time or full time work

> indicate any special qualifications you have for the position

Q: How do hospitals handle unsolicited resumes ?

A: In most instances, they are routed to either the personnel department or to the head of the appropriate unit. Many organizations keep these resumes on file for up to one year. Others will interview applicants for future, as well as current, openings.

The following steps will help you develop a professional nursing resume.

1. **CHOOSE A FORMAT**

   Evaluate the three basic resume formats
   and choose the one that is best for you.

2. **PLAN THE CONTENT**

   Determine what information you will include
   and what information you will omit.

3. **TAKE AN INVENTORY OF YOUR SKILLS**

   Complete a job inventory sheet for each
   position you have held.

4. **DEVELOP SKILL DESCRIPTIONS**

   Write statements about your skills that
   emphasize your accomplishments and the
   results they have produced.

5. **WRITE THE FIRST DRAFT**

   Write a "rough" draft of the content of your
   resume and review for accuracy and completeness.

6. **WRITE THE FINAL DRAFT**

   Polish your resume.

7. **PRODUCE YOUR RESUME**

   Develop a good layout, type the material,
   select the appropriate paper, reproduce
   the resume.

8. **WRITE THE COVER LETTER**

   Produce a cover letter that will make the
   recipient want to read your resume.

9. **CHECK YOUR RESUME AND COVER LETTER**

   Review resume and cover letter for accuracy
   and completeness.

STEP 1 – CHOOSE A FORMAT

There are three basic resume formats. They include the following:

o chronological

o functional

o combination of the two

Chronological. The chronological resume lists your work experience and educational history in reverse chronological order – e.g., the most recent first. Your job experience and education are highlighted with brief descriptions. The chronological resume is probably the most widely used format.

Look at the example provided of the chronological resume on page 10.

Functional. The functional resume organizes your experience according to skill categories, not according to chronology.

Look at the example provided of the functional resume on page 12.

Combination. This format is just what the name indicates. Categories are a combination of skills and chronological work history.

Review the example provided of the combination format on page 14.

Chronological Resume

Jean Redmond
223 Main Street
Washington PA 66901
(417) 128-7521

PROFESSIONAL EXPERIENCE:

1981 - Present   Staff Nurse, Washington Hospital,
                                        Washington, PA.

                                        As a team member on a 35-bed surgical
                                        unit, was responsible for:

                                        - providing care to pre- and post-
                                          operative patients,

                                        - developing methods to assess the
                                          quality of care on the unit,

                                        - instructing patients and their
                                          families in proper at-home care
                                          techniques.

1980-1981   Nursing Assistant, Clairmount Hospital,
                                        Pittsburgh, PA.

                                        Worked full-time for two summers in an
                                        adult surgical unit. Performed such
                                        duties as:

                                        - assisting with physical care of
                                          pre- and post-operative patients,

                                        - developing a program for other
                                          student nurse interns in patient
                                          care,

                                        - recommending efficiency steps to
                                          reduce reporting duplications by
                                          more than 15%.

EDUCATION:

1985   BSN, Washington College, Washington, PA.
                                        (Graduated in top 10% of my class)

1981   AA, Western Pennsylvania College,
                                        Pittsburgh, PA (Graduated with a 3.8
                                        out of possible 4.0 GPA)

HONORS: A.M. Hill Scholarship awarded through
                                             Western Pennsylvania College for pro-
                                             mising students in Nursing, 1981.

                                             "Nursing Student of the Year" award
                                             in 1984 for outstanding achievement.

PROFESSIONAL MEMBERSHIPS:

1981 - Present   American Nurses Association,
                                             Pennsylvania Chapter

1984   Sigma Theta Tau, Alpha Beta Chapter
                                             (Honorary society in nursing)

PROFESSIONAL LICENSE: Pennsylvania RN# 23818

Functional Resume

Mary R. Jenkins
254 Oak Street
Chicago, Illinois 60601

(312) 888-0886

SIGNIFICANT QUALIFICATIONS:

ADMINISTRATION

Served as a high-level nursing administrator in several active health care institutions.

Reorganized staffing and scheduling procedures to improve patient care delivery while decreasing nursing department costs by 20%.

Developed the Nursing Practice Audit that has been adopted by at least seven other area hospitals.

FISCAL MANAGEMENT

Implemented successful strategies to increase recruitment and retention of nursing staff.

Instituted a decentralized budgetary procedure that decreased nursing costs by 22%.

EDUCATION

Established active collaborative role with four local colleges and universities.

Initiated continuing education and other staff development programs.

PROFESSIONAL EXPERIENCE:

Mendall State Hospital, Ames, Iowa
    Executive Director of Nursing   1983 - Present
    Assistant Director of Nursing   1981 - 1983

St. Petronille Hospital, Davenport, Iowa
    Director of Staff Development   1977 - 1981

Freeman Medical Center, Annapolis, MD
    Head Nurse   1975 - 1977

EDUCATION:

MSN Iowa State University, Ames, Iowa, 1981, with honors.

BSN Iowa State University, Ames, Iowa, 1977, with honors.

PROFESSIONAL AFFILIATIONS:

American Hospital Association, Council on Nursing

American Society for Nursing Service Administrators,
Vice President (1983-1985)

National League for Nursing

Combination Resume

Lynne Stauffer
4718 Hamilton Street
San FRancisco, CA 47113
(415) 277-0008

SUMMARY OF QUALIFICATIONS:

ANA Certified Family Nurse Practitioner with expertise in health care
management . . . Joint Practice with two physicians . . . Experience in
administering health care in an outpatient setting . . . Adjunct Assistant
Professor at University of California, San Francisco, preceptor for masters
nursing students and frequent guest lecturer . . . Consultant to nursing
journals and consultant to seven hospitals . . . Experienced researcher.

PROFESSIONAL EXPERIENCE:

1980 - Present

Joint practice with Drs. Ronald Mays
and Pauline Smith, San Francisco, CA.

- Manage health care for families
  in office and at home.

- Conduct health classes for patients
  and families.

- Develop pertinent educational materials
  in such areas as family planning, diabetes,
  cancer prevention, and heart disease.

1981 - Present

Adjunct Assistant Professor, UCSF,
San Francisco, CA.

- Preceptor for masters students in
  Family Nurse Practitioner Program.

- Coordinator of patient care and
  student evaluations.

- Frequent guest lecturer in masters
  program.

EDUCATION:

MS   San Jose State University, San Jose, California, 1980.

BSN Marymount College, Rochester, New York, 1977.

CERTIFICATION:

Nursing Administration, American Nurses Association

Family Nurse Practioner, American Nurses Association

LICENSES

New York RN # 19876   California RN # 35353   14

Choosing the Best Format. Which is the best format for you? The best way to decide is to look at the advantages and disadvantages of each format.

Chronological Resume

    o   Advantages

        This format allows you to:

        - document continuous work activity
          within the nursing field

        - readily highlight career advancement

        - focus on specific jobs and functions

    o   Disadvantages

        This format is **not recommended** if one or more of these situations applies to you:

        - you have had many jobs within
          a short period of time – that is,
          if you have held several jobs for
          one year or less

        - you want to change your career
          objectives

        - you have had the same nursing
          responsibilities in several different
          positions

        - you are returning to nursing after
          a lengthy absence

Functional Resume

o   Advantages

   This format allows you to:

     - concentrate on your accomplish-
       ments, not on the time you spent
       in each position

     - tell how well you performed your
       job

     - minimize or maximize various
       aspects of your career

     - alter your career objectives

     - present yourself in the best light
       after returning to nursing from a
       lengthy absence

o   Disadvantages

   This format also presents certain problems,
   because

     - it is more difficult to show your
       accomplishments in relation to
       your job experience

Combination Resume

o Advantages

This format

- allows you to merge the chronological and functional approaches into one format

- can be a strong selling tool for someone who wants to emphasize both accomplishments and career steps

o Disadvantages

This format also presents some problems, because,

- as with the functional resume, it is more difficult to show given accomplishments in relation to your job experience

- it may be more difficult to organize and write a concise, effective combination resume

STEP 2 - PLAN THE CONTENT

Planning the content of your resume is an extremely important step. It is here that you will determine what information should be conveyed in order to make the kind of impression needed to get that first critical interview.

WHAT TO INCLUDE. Regardless of the type of resume you develop - chronological, functional, or combination - there is certain information you want to include. There is also certain information you **don't** want to include.

Here is the basic information that almost every recruiter or potential employer must know in order to decide if you are a good candidate for the job.

Vital Statistics. Your resume must include your name, address (including zip code), and home telephone number (including area code). You should also indicate your current nursing license number if you have one.

Job Objective. A "Job Objective" statement, while widely used in business, is not as common in nursing. This is because your past professional experience and education play a large part in determining your next career step. Furthermore, if you are applying for a specific, advertised nursing position, a job objective is not required.

There are, however, a few instances in which a "Job Objective" is useful:

o   for entry-level positions - without previous professional experience, it may not otherwise be apparent what job you are seeking

o   when changing direction within nursing, such as moving from staff to management positions, or when moving from a hospital job to a position in another type of facility or environment

o   to identify specific consulting positions

Professional Background. This section answers the crucial question: do you have the right experience for the job? This is the section that most people who evaluate your resume will look at first. Unless you are seeking an entry-level position, this section should take up about two-thirds of your resume.

The recruiter wants to learn two things from your professional background. First, where you have been, the positions you have held, the tasks you have performed and the responsibilities you have handled. Second, the recruiter wants to learn about your accomplishments. Did you initiate positive changes, increase efficiency, improve patient care in specific ways or accomplish any other measurable feats?

An important key to an effective resume is to present your professional experience not simply in terms of the tasks you **performed**, but in terms of **accomplishments** realized. Later in this book, we will show you how to stress your accomplishments.

Education. These guidelines should be followed when presenting your educational background:

o   List your most recent degrees first

o   For each degree, give the date when it was earned and the institution that granted it

o   Indicate any honors, scholarships, or awards you received at each institution

o   Indicate any degrees you anticipate receiving in the near future

o   List under "Additional Education" any certificates that did not lead to a degree, as well as conferences and workshops attended

o   Develop a separate section for "Certification." List the most recent certification first.

o   List any articles, books, or pamphlets that you have written in a "Publications" section. Publication experience is particularly important when you are seeking a teaching or consulting position.

Extracurricular Activities. With two exceptions, it is not recommended that you include a section on "Extracurricular Activities." The two exceptions are:

o   for the beginning nurse

o   for nurses returning to their profession after a long absence

In both cases, it is helpful to include activities where you demonstrated organization, managerial, or any nursing-related skills.

★ **WHAT TO LEAVE OUT.** The information that you should **not** include in your resume is:

Date. Because you want your resume always to be current, never date it.

Personal Data. Do not list physical description, health or marital status, race, religion, age, sex, or political affiliation. Do not include a photo unless one is specifically requested.

Salary Requirements. Mentioning salary in a resume usually works against you. The time to discuss salary is after you have been offered the job, not before. If a salary history is requested, present it in your cover letter.

Availability. It is unnecessary to put "available immediately" on your resume. Why apply today for a job you can't start for another six months?

References. You not only should **not** include
the names of your references, you do not
need to include the phrase, "References available
upon request." The time to offer references
is when they are requested, not before.

Reasons for Leaving a Job. Whether you
left any job for positive or negative reasons,
the place to explain why is during the interview,
not in the resume.

ADDITIONAL GUIDELINES. The following
"Dos and Don'ts" will help you write a better
resume:

o Be brief and to the point. Stick to
   the facts. Never use four words to
   express what can be said in two words.

o Avoid using the word "I." As the resume
   is obviously about you, you do not need
   to mention yourself in the first person
   unless it is awkward to leave it out.

o Keep a businesslike, straightforward
   tone.

o Keep your sentences short and concise.

o Start as many sentences as possible
   with an active word.

o Stress your accomplishments, but do so
   diplomatically. Maybe you did "prevent
   every nurse I supervised from walking
   off the job by instituting needed reforms,"
   but say it diplomatically. For example,
   "instituted new training program that
   reduced turnover by 40% among the nurses
   I supervised."

o Don't mention anything blatantly negative.
   The place to handle that is during the
   interview.

o Check your resume for wording, grammar,
   spelling, and construction. Then have an
   associate double check it for you.

The third step in the process for producing a professional resume is to take an inventory of your skills and accomplishments. This inventory will:

- help you focus on the skills and accomplishments you demonstrated in each position you have held

- enable you to prioritize easily the most important – and more marketable – of these skills

- form a solid foundation for that next important step – developing skill phrases

- become part of the important data bank for your resume

Job Inventory Form. On the next page, you will find a Job Inventory Form. Fill out a separate form for **every** position you have held during the past ten years.

When completing your Job Inventory Form, take into account the following guidelines:

- Start with your most recent position.

- For each position, write down at least five activities you performed and the positive results you achieved. You **don't** need to prioritize the activities at this point.

- If you can't think of five items, write down three or four – you will recall more items later.

- Don't fabricate – but do give yourself credit where it's due.

- Don't worry about how it sounds as you write – just get it down on paper.

- You may use the first person (I) form when completing your inventory form.

JOB INVENTORY FORM

JOB TITLE

ORGANIZATION NAME

DATES OF EMPLOYMENT

What Specific Activities Did You Perform?	What Positive Result Did You Achieve?
1.	1.
2.	2.
3.	3.
4.	4.
5.	5.

A Sample Form. On the following page is
a sample Job Inventory Form for Mary Hill,
currently a relief charge nurse who is seeking
a position as permanent charge nurse.

The Job Inventory Form shown on the next
page is for Mary's most recent position as
relief charge nurse. Mary will complete
a Job Inventory Form for every job she's
held over the last ten years.

Note that whenever possible, Mary has backed
up her accomplishments with specific results.
For example, "I increased participation in
the program by 25%."

Whenever you can, you should cite percentages
and numbers that demonstrate positive results.
This will require you to do some research
and analysis, but the results are well worth
the effort. If you cannot obtain exact figures,
you can qualify your figures with words like
"approximately," "around," or "almost."

Recent Graduates. For recent nursing graduates
with little or no professional experience,
certain guidelines need to be followed.

If you are a recent graduate, you need to
develop a **Job Inventory Form** for each job
you have held – whether or not it was nursing
related.

With these jobs, you should focus on the
skills and accomplishments that can be applied
to nursing. For example, if you were a sales
clerk in a women's clothing store, a specific
activity you performed might be: "selling
clothing." The positive result of this activity
might be: "increased sales in my department
by 37% within the first 90 days." Obviously,
your goal is to identify activities, skills, and
results that depict you as hardworking, enthu-
siastic, creative, and able to show initiative.
Most recruiters will easily see that these
are real assets for a nurse to have.

JOB INVENTORY FORM

JOB TITLE

ORGANIZATION NAME

DATES OF EMPLOYMENT

What Specific Activities Did You Perform?	What Positive Results Did You Achieve?
1. I educated families and patients about better health habits.	1. I increased participation in the program by 25%.
2. Instituted a Patient Audit program to improve patient care.	2. Was able to verify objectively that patient care improved because of this program.
3. Made staff assignments	3. Because our staff was working more effectively and efficiently, use of on-call personnel reduced by 25%.
4. Served as communication liaison between staff and administration.	4. Because of more open communication, employee satisfaction increased on annual survey and absenteeism decreased by 23% among nurses reporting to me.
5. Maintained files and records on patients and nurses I was responsible for.	5. Reduced amount of time needed to maintain files by 15%.

You should treat all nursing-related and community volunteer jobs as a regular paid job.
Fill out a Job Inventory Form for each position.
Again, the idea is to focus on activities and
positive results that make you marketable.

**If You're Returning to Nursing After a Lengthy
Absence.** If you are returning to nursing
after an absence of five years or more, you
should complete a Job Inventory Form for
each position you held in the ten years **prior**
to your layoff.

STEP 4 – DEVELOP SKILL DESCRIPTIONS

Once your Job Inventory Forms are completed, you are ready to write the first draft of your resume. To help you do that, you should develop a series of "action" words and phrases that describe your accomplishments in vivid, positive, concise language.

The objective here is to supply you with the dynamic words and phrases you want to use when describing your abilities in the "work experience" section of your resume. By taking the time now to develop such words and phrases, you make writing your first draft much easier. When you have completed this step, you will have a list of phrases for four or five tasks and accomplishments for **each** position you have held.

To illustrate how it works, let's look again at Mary Hill's Job Inventory Form for her position as relief charge nurse. For each specific activity she performed, she also listed a positive result she achieved.

For example, Mary wrote on her Job Inventory Form: "I educated families and patients about better health habits. . . I increased participation in the program by 25%." Mary's goal is to condense all of this information into 10 to 15 dynamic, attention-getting words. She rewrote this information to read: "Conducted a patient/family 'Better Health' course and increased participation by 25%."

There are several things to note about Mary's rewrite. First, whenever possible, she started a phrase with an action word, such as "conducted, directed, established." She tied what she **did** to what she **accomplished.** For example, what Mary **did** was "conduct a course." What she **accomplished** was "increased participation by 25%."

When developing your phrases, keep in mind that your objective is to reflect as **active, positive, dynamic** an image as possible.

To do this, you should:

o **Be specific.** Generalizations have little meaning, specific information creates an impact. For example:

General: Served in a supervisory role over a staff of 12.

Specific: Supervised a med/surge staff of seven RNs and five LVNs.

General: Maintained high academic performance throughout my college career.

Specific: Graduated in top 10% of my college class.

o **Give results whenever possible.** For example:

Don't say: Successfully administered department's paper work.

Do say: Increased administrative efficiency by 20%.

o **Be concise.** You want to telegraph information in a readable fashion. For example:

Don't say: I was placed in charge of two rehab units consisting of 10 nurses.

Do say: Supervised two rehab units with staff of 10 RNs.

o **Use action words and descriptive phrases.** For example:

Don't say: I assisted in orientation of new staff members.

Do say: Oriented as many as 10 new charge nurses each month.

Don't say: My principle duties as head
nurse involved supervising staff of 7
emergency room nurses in a 50-bed unit.

Do say: Supervised a staff of 7 RNs in
a 50-bed emergency room unit.

As a general rule, if your resume demonstrates
ten specific accomplishments, you have a
strong resume.

If you have trouble developing phrases that
describe your accomplishments, try completing
the following statements:

I organized . . .

I created . . .

I established . . .

I revamped . . .

I developed . . .

I supervised . . .

I strengthened . . .

I instituted . . .

I reduced . . .

I saved . . .

I improved . . .

I coordinated . . .

WORD LIST

Here is a list of words that will help you create a positive impact.

accelerate	create	initiate	recommend
accomplish	decide	innovate	reconcile
achieve	define	inspect	record
act	delegate	install	recruit
activate	demonstrate	institute	rectify
adapt	design	instruct	re-design
adjust	detail	integrate	reduce
administer	determine	interpret	reinforce
advertise	develop	interview	relate
advise	devise	investigate	renew
affect	direct	invent	reorganize
analyze	distribute	launch	report
anticipate	draft	lead	represent
apply	edit	maintain	research
approach	educate	manage	resolve
approve	effect	market	revamp
arrange	eliminate	mediate	review
assemble	encourage	merchandize	revise
assess	enlarge	moderate	scan
assign	enlist	modify	schedule
assist	establish	monitor	screen
attain	estimate	motivate	select
author	evaluate	negotiate	serve
budget	examine	obtain	set up
build	exchange	operate	simplify
calculate	execute	organize	solve
catalog	expand	originate	solicit
chair	expedite	participate	speak
clarify	facilitate	perceive	staff
collaborate	familiarize	perform	standardize
communicate	forecast	persuade	stimulate
compare	formulate	pinpoint	summarize
complete	generate	plan	strategize
conceive	govern	present	streamline
conceptualize	guide	preside	strengthen
conciliate	handle	problem-solve	structure
conduct	hire	process	supervise
confer	identify	produce	survey
consult	implement	program	synthesize
contract	improve	promote	systematize
control	increase	propose	teach
cooperate	index	provide	team-build
coordinate	influence	publicize	train
counsel	inform	publish	transmit

ACTION PHRASES

Below are additional action phrases that you can use when describing your abilities and accomplishments.

Competence. When you want to stress your competence, you might use phrases such as:

creative	technical competence in
strength in	know-how
ability to	aptitude for
thoroughly trained	first hand knowledge of
mastered	practical approach to
well grounded	performance oriented
proficient	proven track record in
effective in	comprehensive knowledge of
capacity for	results-oriented
adept at	thorough understanding of

Ability to Handle Details. If you want to stress your ability to handle details, you can say:

detail-minded	methodical
pay attention to detail	careful
systematic	orderly
precise	accurate
well organized	efficient
get things done	use follow-through

Responsibility. Words and phrases that indicate your desire to assume responsibility include:

capacity to	accept responsibility
meet deadlines	tackle a job
energetic	perform well under pressure
vigorous	self-motivated
enthusiastic	persistent
troubleshooter in	show a commitment to

Management Ability. Words or phrases indicating management ability include:

headed	people-oriented skills
took charge	administered
decision maker	authority over
closely supervised	directed
high-level supervisory skills	leadership ability
ranking member of	developed subordinates
spearheaded	in charge of
willing to take the initiative	

General. Words and phrases that are generally useful include:

self-disciplined	like an environment that
self-reliant	necessary ingredients for
self-confident	conscientious
diplomatic	enjoy getting involved with
discreet	good back-up for
tactful	persuasive
success-oriented	understand priorities
aptitude for	

STEP 5 – WRITE THE FIRST DRAFT

Your next step is to write a first, rough draft of
your resume. Your goal here is **not** to have a
finished product. Rather, your goal is to decide
on a format, decide what material will be included,
and then put this material down on paper.

To help you do this, we will show you the first
draft of Mary Hill's resume. Here are the steps
Mary took to complete this draft.

Step One. Choosing a Format. Mary chooses
the chronological resume format for these reasons:

o She has no employment gaps over the
   last several years . A chronological
   resume highlights this kind of continuous
   work history

o Each position she's held has had more responsibility than her previous position.
   A chronological resume highlights this
   fact.

Step Two. Planning the Content. Mary decides
to include the following information and to present
it in this order:

o Vital Statistics (Name, Address, Phone Number)

o Professional Experience

o Education

o Professional Organizations

o Awards

o Publications

o Nursing Registration Number

Step Three. Take a Skills Inventory. We already
saw how Mary completed her Job Inventory Form
for her most recent position, that of relief charge
nurse. On the following pages, you will see how
she completes the Job Inventory Forms for her
previous two positions.

Step Four. Develop Skill Descriptions. Mary's next
step is to develop short action statements that
put her skills and accomplishments into concise,
dynamic language.

Mary goes back to her Job Inventory Form and
reworks her description of activities she performed
and her accomplishments.

Her rewrites look like this:

Job Inventory Form

Position: Relief Charge Nurse/Critical Care

What Specific Activities Did You Perform?	**What Positive Results Did You Achieve?**
1. I educated families and patients about better health habits.	1. I increased participation in the program by 25%.

Rewrite

Conducted a patient/family "Better Health" course and
increased participation by 25%.

Job Inventory Form

What Specific Activities Did You Perform?	**What Positive Results Did You Achieve?**
2. Instituted a Patient Audit program to improve patient care.	2. Was able to verify objectively that patient care improved because of this program.

Rewrite

Instituted a "Patient Audit" program that improved the
level of patient care.

Job Inventory Form

What Specific Activities Did You Perform?

What Positive Results Did You Achieve?

3. Made staff assignments.

3. Because our staff was working more effectively and efficiently, use of on-call personnel was reduced by 25%.

Rewrite

Reduced the use of on-call personnel by 25% by improving efficiency of regular staffing.

Job Inventory Form

What Specific Activities Did You Perform?

What Positive Results Did You Achieve?

4. Served as communication liaison between staff and administration.

4. Because of more open communication, employee satisfaction increased on annual survey and absenteeism decreased by 23% among nurses reporting to me.

Rewrite

Initiated better communication between administration and my staff which helped increase employee satisfaction and decrease absenteeism by 23%.

Job Inventory Form

What Specific Activities Did You Perform?

What Positive Results Did You Achieve?

5. Maintained files and records on patients and nurses I was responsible for.

5. Reduced amount of time needed to maintain files by 15%.

Rewrite

Reduced file maintenance time by 15%.

Position: Supervisor in Nursing Department

Job Inventory Form

What Specific Activities Did You Perform?

What Positive Results Did You Achieve?

1. Initiated new concepts for patient care delivery.

1. We were able to reduce average length of stay by 15%.

Rewrite

Instituted new patient care delivery techniques that reduced average length of stay by 15%.

Job Inventory Form

What Specific Activities Did You Perform?

What Positive Results Did You Achieve?

2. Made scheduling assignments for seven nursing personnel; delegated responsibilities.

2. Because of increased efficiency in scheduling, we were able to reduce overtime by 40%.

Rewrite

Decreased amount of overtime by 40% through better scheduling and delegation of activities.

Job Inventory Form

What Specific Activities Did You Perform?

3. Managed conflict resolution.

What Positive Results Did You Achieve?

3. Because I was able to effectively resolve employee conflicts, employee satisfaction increased on annual survey and work time lost due to conflict among personnel decreased by 50%.

Rewrite

Increased employee satisfaction and decreased time lost due to conflict among personnel by 50% through more effective conflict resolution.

Job Inventory Form

What Specific Activities Did You Perform?

4. Streamlined and revised hospital's policies and procedures as they pertained to our unit.

What Positive Results Did You Achieve?

4. This was the first revision to the procedures in five years. Hospital administrator praised the job as one that helped the hospital run more efficiently.

Rewrite

Initiated first reform of hospital procedures and policies to occur in five years. Administrator said it made the hospital run more efficiently.

Job Inventory Form

What Specific Activities Did You Perform?

5. Made important recommendations for my unit's budget.

What Positive Results Did You Achieve?

5. Because I was able to provide
   more realistic cost projections than
   what we had before, we were able
   to keep expenditures to previous
   year's level.

Rewrite

Developed recommendations that eliminated need to increase
unit budget.

Position: Education Coordinator for Planned Parenthood

Job Inventory Form

What Specific Activities Did You Perform?

1. Planned and created entire
   program.

What Positive Results Did You Achieve?

1. Because I upgraded the course
   content, we increased participation
   by 20% over the previous year.

Rewrite

Planned, created, and upgraded program that resulted in 20%
increase in participation.

Job Inventory Form

What Specific Activities Did You Perform?

2. I hired, trained, and directed
   three assistants.

What Positive Results Did You Achieve?

2. The reaction to my staff was very
   positive. Participants related well
   to them and my supervisor said this
   was one of the best program staffs
   she had seen in ten years.

Rewrite

Hired, trained, and directed staff of three that was rated
by hospital management as one of the best in the past ten years.

Job Inventory Form

What Specific Activities Did You Perform?	**What Positive Results Did You Achieve?**
3. Scheduled classes.	3. Because I used greater flexibility in arranging schedule, classes averaged a 90% attendance rate.

Rewrite

Developed a flexible class schedule that helped maintain a
90% attendance rate.

Job Inventory Form

What Specific Activities did You Perform?	**What Positive Results Did You Achieve?**
4. I organized a special class for the learning disabled.	4. This was the first time we had participation by the learning disabled in this program.

Rewrite

Organized a first-ever class for the learning disabled.

Job Inventory Form

What Specific Activities Did You Perform?	**What Positive Results Did You Achieve?**
5. Used input from participants and staff to modify next year's course.	5. By further improving the course, we increased enrollment by 10% in the following year's program.

Rewrite

Utilized teachers' and participants' input to improve second year's program and increase enrollment by 10%.

The First Draft. With these steps completed, Mary is ready to write her first draft. Look at the following page for an example.

After you write your first draft, your next step is to put your resume away for two or three days. You will then be ready to write your second draft.

MARY HILL
360 S. Main street
Glen Ellyn, Illinois 60137
(312) 469-3403

PROFESSIONAL EXPERIENCE

Relief Charge Nurse/Critical Care
Elmhurst Hospital
Elmhurst, Illinois

1983 - Present

  1. Conducted a patient/family "Better Health" course and increased
      participation by 25%.

  2. Instituted a "Patient Audit" program that improved the level of
      patient care.

  3. Reduced use of on-call personnel by 25% by improving efficiency
      of regular staffing.

  4. Initiated better communication between administration and my
      staff which helped increase employee satisfaction and decrease
      absenteeism by 23%.

  5. Reduced file maintenance time by 15%.

Supervisor in Nursing Department
Oak Park Hospital
Oak Park, Illinois

1981 - 1983

  1. Instituted new patient care delivery techniques that reduced
      average length of stay by 15%.

  2. Decreased amount of overtime by 40% through better scheduling
      and delegation of activities.

  3. Increased employee satisfaction and decreased time lost due to
      conflict among personnel by 50% through more effective conflict
      resolution.

  4. Initiated first reform of hospital procedures and policies to
      occur in five years. Administrator said it made the hospital
      run more efficiently.

  5. Developed recommendations that eliminated need to increase
      unit budget.

Hill, Mary Continued

Education Coordinator for Planned Parenthood
West Suburban Hospital
Winfield, Illinois

1979 - 1981

1. Planned, created, and upgraded program that resulted in 20%
    increase in participation.

2. Hired, trained, and directed staff of three that was rated
    by hospital management as one of the best in the past ten years.

3. Developed a flexible class schedule that helped maintain a
    90% attendance rate.

4. Organized a first-ever class for the learning disabled.

5. Utilized teachers' and participants' input to improve second
    year's program and increase enrollment by 10%.

EDUCATION

B.S.N., Illinois State University, Normal, Illinois, 1981.
Graduated in top 15% of my class.

PROFESSIONAL ORGANIZATIONS

Critical Care Nursing Association
American Nurses Association
Illinois Nurses Association

AWARDS

Sigma Theta Tau (Nursing Honor Society), 1980-1981.
Elected to "League for Outstanding Nursing Service," 1983.

PUBLICATIONS

"Developing An Effective Planned Parenthood Program," Nursing Outlook, 1981.

"Improving Staff Efficiency," American Journal of Nursing, 1983.

PROFESSIONAL NURSING LICENSE

Illinois RN # 8976-G

STEP 6 – WRITE THE FINAL DRAFT

After you have allowed the first draft of your
resume to "hibernate" for a few days, you are
ready to look at it again and refine the text.

Basically, you will concentrate on the following
four areas when producing your second draft:

o **Language**

> You want the descriptions of your
> job responsibilities and accomplish-
> ments to be concise, clear, and
> powerfully written.

o **Content**

> You want to be sure to eliminate
> any extraneous information and/or
> add any important information
> that was left out.

o **Organization**

> You need to prioritize your job
> responsibilities and accomplishments
> so that the most important appear
> first.

o **Tone**

> You want the style of your language
> to be light, not bureaucratic or
> academic. You also want it to be
> professional, not familiar or flip.

With these four points in mind, let's look at how
Mary Hill improves her first draft.

Language. After reviewing the action phrases
that describe her job responsibilities and accomplishments, Mary decides that some of them
could be written better. On the following page
you will see phrases from her first draft and
the rewrites for her second draft. Can you determine why the rewrite is an improvement over
the first version?

First Draft	**Second Draft**
1. Conducted a patient/family "Better Health course and increased participation by 25%.	1. Directed a patient/family "Better Health" course and increased participation by 25%.
2. Instituted a "Patient Audit" program that improved the level of patient care.	2. Improved level of patient care by instituting a "Patient Audit" program.
3. Reduced use of on-call personnel by 25% by improving efficiency of regular staffing.	3. The statement remains the same.
4. Initiated better communication between administration and my staff which helped increase employee satisfaction and decrease absenteeism by 23%.	4. Initiated better communication between administration and staff. Increased employee satisfaction and decreased absenteeism by 23%.
5. Reduced file maintenance time by 15%.	5. This statement remains the same.
6. Instituted new patient care delivery techniques that reduced average length of stay by 15%.	6. Reduced average length of stay by 15% through improved patient care delivery techniques.
7. Decreased amount of overtime by 40% through better scheduling and delegation of activities.	7. This statement remains the same.
8. Increased employee satisfaction and decreased time lost due to conflict among personnel by 50% through more effective conflict resolution.	8. Improved management of conflict resolution that helped reduce time lost due to conflict by 50%.
9. Initiated first reform of hospital procedures and policies to occur in five years. Administrator said it made the hospital run more efficiently.	9. Initiated first reform of departmental procedures to occur in five years. Hospital administrator said: "These changes make the hospital function more efficiently."
10. Developed recommendations that eliminated need to increase unit budget.	10. Eliminated need to increase unit budget by developing cost-saving recommendations.

First Draft

11. Planned, created, and upgraded program that resulted in 20% increase in participation.

12. Hired, trained, and directed staff of three that was rated by hospital management as one of the best in the past ten years.

13. Developed a flexible class schedule that helped maintain a 90% attendance rate.

14. Organized a first-ever class for the learning disabled.

15. Utilized teachers' and participants' input to improve second year's program and increase enrollment by 10%.

Second Draft

11. Planned, created, and upgraded program that saw a 20% increase in participation.

12. Hired, trained, and directed staff of three rated by hospital administration as "one of the best in the past ten years."

13. Developed a flexible class schedule that helped produce a 90% attendance rate.

14. This statement remains the same.

15. Improved second year program and increased its enrollment by 10%.

Content. After making these changes, Mary
looks at her resume and asks herself two questions.
First, "have I included any information that is
unnecessary?" Second, "have I omitted any important information?"

In answer to question one, Mary sees some information she can consolidate or eliminate. In her
position as "Education Coordinator for Planned
Parenthood," for example, one of her accomplishments was that she "Improved second year program
and increased enrollment by 10%." Mary now
decides that this is not particularly meaningful
to the job for which she is now applying. So,
she decides to eliminate it.

For her position as relief charge nurse, she
decides that the statement, "Initiated better
communication between administration and staff"
is too subjective to be very meaningful. Consequently, she decides to eliminate it. But, she
retains the strong, objective statement: "Decreased absenteeism by 23%. "

In answer to her second question, Mary also decides that for each position shown on her resume,
she should add a brief job description. This will
enable the prospective employer to see at a
glance the full range of that position's responsibilities. So, for her position as relief charge
nurse, she writes: "Performed all charge nurse
duties for an active 25 bed critical care unit
at a top-rated hospital facility."

For her position as a supervisor in the nursing
department, Mary adds the statement: "Managed
a staff of seven RNs and two LVNs in a 30
bed rehab unit at a 300 bed hospital."

For her position as educational coordinator for
Planned Parenthood, Mary adds the statement:
"Assumed complete responsibility for development and implementation of a program that
has over 750 participants annually."

When determining what information should be
cut and what should be added, keep in mind what

is important to the position you are seeking.
By eliminating unimportant material, you make
the remaining statements much stronger and
more meaningful.

Organization. In reviewing her resume draft,
Mary asks herself: "Are my job responsibilities
and accomplishments listed so that the most
important are shown first?" Again, she wants
to highlight skills and responsibilities that are
significant for the job she's seeking. For the
results of how she reorganized her material,
compare the order in which her responsibilities
are shown in her first draft to the order in which
they appear in the second draft.

Note the following about Mary's rewritten phrases:

o   Several of them were written so well the
    first time that Mary didn't need to rewrite
    them.

o   Her changes generally fell into these categories:

    - Making statements more positive. In ex-
       ample # 2, the rewrite reads: "Improved
       level of patient care by instituting a "Patient
       Audit program." This rewrite puts the
       result of the action – improved patient care –
       at the beginning of the statement rather
       than at the end where it was in the first
       draft.

    - Inserting direct quotes – as in examples
       # 9 and # 12 – makes these statements much
       stronger and more credible.

    - Strengthening the language. Instead of
       "instituted **new** patient care delivery tech-
       niques," the rewrite of # 6 reads "improved
       patient care delivery techniques."

    - Dividing lengthy statements into two sen-
       tences for greater clarity.

    - Making statements shorter and more concise
       wherever possible.

Tone. Mary reviews the resume for tone. She
sees that the tone is direct and professional.
She doesn't use the word "I" or make flip statements.
She has not used any "buzz" words or abbrevia-
tions that might not be understood. Consequently,
Mary decides that her resume passes the test
of presenting a good, professional tone.

The Final Draft. Once she has completed her
changes, Mary's resume is ready for the final
draft. A sample of this final version appears
on the following pages.

Before you finalize your resume text, it is suggested
that you

- o   put it away again for several days

- o   rewrite it one more time and make
       final corrections

- o   ask friends and associates to critique it

MARY HILL
360 S. Main Street
Glen Ellyn, Illinois 60137
(312) 469-3403

PROFESSIONAL EXPERIENCE

1983 - Present   Relief Charge Nurse/Critical Care
                         Elmhurst Hospital
                         Elmhurst, Illinois

                         Performed all charge nurse duties for
                         25-bed critical care unit at a top-rated
                         facility.

                         Significant accomplishments include:

                         - Reduced use of on-call personnel by 25%
                           by improving efficiency of regular staffing.

                         - Improved level of patient care by instituting
                           a "Patient Audit" program.

                         - Reduced file maintenance time by 15%.

                         - Directed a patient/family "Better Health" course
                           and increased participation by 25%.

                         - Decreased absenteeism on unit by 23%.

1981 - 1983   Supervisor in Nursing Department
                         Oak Park Hospital
                         Oak Park, Illinois

                         Managed a staff of seven RNs and two LVNs in a 30-bed
                         rehab unit at a 300-bed hospital.

                         - Decreased amount of overtime by 40% through better
                           scheduling and delegation of activities.

                         - Reduced average length of stay by 15% through
                           improved patient care delivery techniques.

                         - Eliminated need to increase unit budget by developing
                           cost-saving recommendations.

                         - Improved management of conflict resolution that
                           helped reduce time lost due to conflict by 50%.

                         - Initiated first reform of departmental procedures
                           to occur in five years. Hospital administrator said:
                           "These changes make the hospital function more
                           efficiently."

Hill, Mary   Continued

1979 - 1981   Education Coordinator for Planned Parenthood
                           West Suburban Hospital
                           Winfield, Illinois

                           Assumed complete responsibility for development
                           and implementation of a program that has over 750
                           participants annually. Accomplishments were

                           - Hired, trained, and directed staff of three, rated
                             by hospital administration as "one of the best
                             in past ten years."

                           - Planned, created, and upgraded program that saw
                             a 20% increase in participation.

                           - Developed a flexible class schedule that helped
                             produce a 90% attendance rate.

                           - Organized a first-ever class for the learning
                             disabled.

EDUCATION

B.S.N., Illinois State University, Normal, Illinois, 1981.
Graduated in top 15% of my class.

PROFESSIONAL ORGANIZATIONS

Critical Care Nursing Association
American Nurses Association
Illinois Nurses Association

AWARDS

Sigma Theta Tau (Nursing Honor Society), 1980-1981.
Elected to "League for Outstanding Nursing Service," 1983.

PUBLICATIONS

"Developing An Effective Planned Parenthood Program," Nursing Outlook, 1981.

"Improving Staff Efficiency," American Journal of Nursing, 1983.

PROFESSIONAL NURSING LICENSE

Illinois RN # 8976-G

STEP 7 – PRODUCE YOUR RESUME

When you are satisfied with the content and writing of your resume, you are ready to produce it.

The way your resume is produced is extremely important. Again, think about the recruiter or potential employer who may be reviewing hundreds of resumes for one position. The resume that looks professional will register a more favorable impression than one that does not.

Here are some guidelines that will help you produce a resume that looks professional.

Planning the Layout. Before you type your resume, decide how it will be laid out. Take a blank piece of paper and pencil in one-inch margins around the entire page. This is now a working model of your actual page. Within the margins, roughly determine how many lines can fit comfortably on the page. Indicate the appropriate title and text blocks and the appropriate space. It is suggested that you put three spaces between each content area.

Your layout will be determined by the resume format you use. The layout for a chronological resume will differ from a functional or combination resume. Look at the examples of the various layout approaches presented on the following pages.

Charlene Jenkins
552 Woodrush Place
Scranton PA 12534
(215) 745-3617

PROFESSIONAL EXPERIENCE

1983 – Present

Senior Nurse Coordinator
Mercy Hospital
Scranton, Pennsylvania

Coordinate all nursing activities for three units
(120 beds) in a 500-bed hospital. Duties include:
- Budget Development for three nursing units.
- Initiation and Administration of hospital's
  first Staff Enhancement Conference.
- Establish performance review system for
  nurses that increased productivity by 18%.
- Chair curriculum committee at Scranton
  College's School of Nursing.

1980 – 1983

Staff Nurse
St. Louis Memorial Hospital
St. Louis, Missouri

Responsible for coordinating and providing
care for two units (75 beds) in a 300-bed
hospital. Was required to:
- Institute time-saving techniques that reduced
  average patient stay by 15%.
- Monitor quality and efficiency of patient care.
- Develop three new continuing education courses
  for first-year staff members
- Increase staff participation in courses by 34%.

Jenkins, Charlene Continued

EDUCATION

M.S.N. Villanova University, College of Nursing,
        Villanova, PA 1980
        Graduated 23rd out of a class of 367

B.S.N. St. Louis University, St. Louis, Missouri 1980
        Maintained a 3.0 grade point average while working 25 hours per week.

PROFESSIONAL ORGANIZATIONS

American Society for Nursing Administration
Association of College Nurses (Past President)

PUBLICATIONS

"The Role of the Nursing Administrator in Adult Health Care," Nursing
Management, 1983.

PROFESSIONAL NURSING LICENSES

Pennsylvania # 33834-H
Missouri # 279JAZ

FUNCTIONAL RESUME

Diane Perry
1113 S. Oak Park Avenue
Takoma Park, MD 37162
(315) 872-6522

SELECTED ACCOMPLISHMENTS

Adult Nurse Practitioner in urban ambulatory care clinic.
Manager of care for more than 150 adult patients.

PHYSICAL EXAM   Proficient in complete physical assessment,
                              including pelvic exam.

LAB SKILLS AND TESTS   Skilled in venipuncture and finger puncture for:
                                Blood culture
                                Gardenella
                                Gram Stains
                                Hematocrit
                                Monilia
                                Monospot
                                Throat culture
                                Urine culture
                                Urine pregnancy test

CLINICAL TESTS   Electrocardiogram, CPR, Pulmonary function test,
                              Stress test

CLIENT EDUCATION   Developed pamphlets for adults on nutrition, low
                              sodium diets, and exercise.

                              Conducted health classes on hypertension, diabetes,
                              and glaucoma.

                              Instructed new nursing staff members in hospital's
                              testing procedures.

Perry, Diane Continued

EDUCATION   MSN Simons University, Lexington, MA   1982
                   BSN University of Vermont, Burlington, VT   1974

PROFESSIONAL EXPERIENCE

Adult Nurse Practitioner   1982 - Present
Towson Hospital, Towson MD

Staff Nurse, Emergency Room   1976 - 1978
Valley Hospital,
Montpellier VT

Public Health Nurse   1974 - 1976
Lehigh Dept of Health
Montpellier VT

PROFESSIONAL MEMBERSHIPS

American Nurses' Association
Maryland Nurses' Association (Program Committee, 1980-82)
Adult Nurses' Practitioners Association

PROFESSIONAL NURSING LICENSES

Massachusetts # 956232-J
Vermont # A2538

COMBINATION RESUME

Janet R. Lansing
2344 Fairview Drive
Costa Mesa CA   95626
(714) 956-9876

SUMMARY OF QUALIFICATIONS

ANA certified oncology specialist . . .Established new oncology unit for
400 bed hospital . . . Developed unit's procedures and policies, recruited
and trained new staff . . . Wrote and taught cancer treatment techniques
for nursing staff of 35 . . . Handled public cancer education courses . . .
Developed seminars for health professionals . . . Instituted more efficient
and comprehensive patient forms, including chemotherapy flow sheet, discharge
instructions, medication records.

PROFESSIONAL EXPERIENCE

Oncology Specialist, Mesa Hills Community Hospital, Mesa Hills, California,
1981 - present.

Nursing Specialist, Lakeview Gardens Convalescent Hospital, Lakeview
Terrace, California, 1978 - 1981.

Unit Coordinator for Hematology/Oncology, Santa Ana Hospital, Santa Ana,
California, 1976 - 1978.

On-call nurse, St. Jude Hospital, Mirada Springs, California, 1974 - 1976.

EDUCATION

AA Degree in Nursing - Mesa Hills College, 1973
Biology of Cancer - University of California, Irvine, 1975
Oncology Nursing - University of California, Irvine 1975

PROFESSIONAL LICENSE   56

California # B483967

Typing your Resume. If you are an excellent typist and have a machine that types a firm, dark, clear impression, you can type your resume yourself. However, there are several advantages to having it typed professionally:

- o you can expect – and demand – a letter-perfect job,

- o you can use a typist who has access to a word processor with typesetting capabilities – a resume that is typeset gives a thoroughly professional impression,

- o by having your resume put into a word processor, you can have additional copies made easily and you can update your resume very quickly.

Printing Your Resume. Once your resume has been typed or typeset, you are ready to have it printed. When doing so, you should:

- o use 20 pound high quality bond paper,

- o stick to white or off-white shades; do not use pastels or other colored papers,

- o do not send a carbon copy or one that has been produced on a mimeograph machine.

For beginning nurses, good xerographed copies are fine. However, for higher level positions, it is suggested that you take your resume and your paper to a copy center and have it printed on an offset press. While it will cost more than putting it through a copy machine, the end result will be crisp and professional looking.

Many job seekers make one of two crucial mistakes when it comes to the cover letter. They either put little effort into producing a good one – or, they don't produce one at all.

You could, of course, send your resume off without a cover letter. But, to make a thoroughly professional presentation, a letter is necessary. A solidly-crafted cover letter can accomplish these things for you:

o   It adds a personal touch. With a few sentences, you can introduce yourself to the potential employer.

o   It tells the recruiter the job for which you are applying. When you consider that a recruiter may be screening candidates for many different positions, this becomes important.

o   It gives you the opportunity to recap your qualifications and state why you are right for the job.

Cover Letter Guidelines. Below are some general rules for you to follow when writing your cover letter.

o   **Keep your letter brief and professional.** It should be no longer than two or three concisely written paragraphs that are organized around three sections: introduction, explanation, and closing.

o   **One good cover letter can be used over and over again.** You simply change the name, hospital or organization, address, and particulars about the job.

o   **Direct the letter to the appropriate person.** Do not address it "To whom it may concern," or "Nurse Recruiter," or "Hospital Administrator." Again, you want to do everything you can to establish good rapport with the person who is reviewing your credentials. Obtain a name by calling the hospital or organization.

o **Open with a strong lead.** Get right to the point. Your opening sentences should create an immediate rapport and establish your professional value. They should answer the questions: "Who are you? What do you want?"

o **Choose your words carefully.** Just as you did with your resume, use strong, action words that convey determination, awareness, eagerness, and professionalism.

o **Close on a positive note.** Just as you opened with an upbeat, confident tone, you should close in a positive way. Don't leave the recruiter in suspense. Say that you would like to get together as soon as possible; or that you would like to set up an appointment; or that you will follow up with a telephone call if you don't hear back within ten days. In other words, make it clear that you will take the initiative if you don't get a response.

Look at the examples of cover letters provided on the following pages.

                                              2323 South Street
                                              New Haven, CT 06516
                                              October 25, 1985

Debra Bradley, RN
Nursing Recruiter
St. Mark's Hospital
1801 Cutrone Drive
New Haven CT 16850

Dear Ms. Bradly:

I am graduating from the University of New Haven, College of Nursing,
with a BSN in May, 1986. I am seeking a staff nurse position in a
pediatric or obstetrical unit.

Enclosed is my resume for your review. I will be happy to forward any
transcripts or other information you need. I will be available for an
interview the week of November 10.

I will call you this Monday to set up a time that is convenient for you.
Thanks again for your consideration.

                              Sincerely,

                              Janice Norris

Comments on Janice Norris' Letter

This letter was not written in response to a specific ad, but is making a general
inquiry about available positions.

Janice took the trouble to find out to whom her letter should be addressed.
This gives her letter greater impact.

While brief, the letter contains all of the necessary information: her background,
position she wants, resume is enclosed, when she can interview, when she will
call to set up an interview, thanks the recruiter for her time and consideration.

3178 Kime Street
Elkhart, Indiana 46514
November 23, 1985

Roxanne J. Smith, RN, MSN
Associate Administrator
West Community Hospital
Elkhart, Indiana 46516

Dear Ms. Smith:

Ms. Judy Johnson, Director of Nursing at Kennedy General Hospital, Gary, suggested that I contact you about the position of Assistant Director of Nursing.

My four years' experience in Nursing Administration as a Clinical Director in a large, urban health center and my academic credentials in nursing administration have prepared me to assume this important position.

Enclosed please find my resume for your review.

I will telephone you in a week to confirm an appointment. Thank you for your time and consideration.

Sincerely,

Stephanie Greene, RN

Comments on Stephanie Greene's Letter

This letter was written at the suggestion of someone who knows the nursing administrator. Because this is important, this reference comes in the first sentence.

The applicant then briefly recaps the experience that is relevant to the position she is seeking.

She says when she will call for an interview.

She thanks the administrator for her time and consideration.

2145 Ford Drive
Alexandria VA 22310
April 4, 1985

Dorothy R. Lane, RN
Commonwealth Hospital
2920 Sunbury Drive
Alexandria VA 22303

Dear Ms. Lane:

I am inquiring about the availability of Family Nurse Practitioner
positions at Commonwealth Hospital.

I am an ANA Certified Family Nurse Practitioner with three years'
experience and broad clinical and laboratory skills. The resume
enclosed describes the scope of my expertise.

I will phone you next week to set up a time when we can meet to discusss
your needs further. Thank you for your help.

Sincerely,

Claudia Ryan, MSN, RN

Comments on Claudia Ryan's Letter

While Claudia is making an unsolicited inquiry, she has taken the time to find
out who should receive her letter and resume.

She indicates the purpose of her letter in the first paragraph and her significant
qualifications in the second paragraph.

She closes by indicating when she will call the nurse recruiter to set up an
interview and thanks the recruiter for her time.

STEP 9 – CHECK YOUR RESUME AND COVER LETTER

Before you send out your resume and cover letter, you should review them in the light of the checklist below. Mark each question with a check in either the "Yes" or "No" box. When you are done, you will know whether or not your material needs more work before it can go to work for you.

APPEARANCE AND FORMAT   YES   NO

Is your resume neatly typed or machine printed?   _____   _____

Is the typing good with no errors, strikeovers, or
obvious erasures?   _____   _____

Does it appear on only one side of each page ?   _____   _____

Is the text neatly centered on the page?   _____   _____

Is the paper of good quality and a white or off-white color? _____   _____

Is the paper no larger than $8\frac{1}{2}$" x 11"?   _____   _____

If reproduced, is the type sharp and clean and the paper
spotless?   _____   _____

Have you used an attractive, business-like type style?
(not script)   _____   _____

Is the print of typewriter size, avoiding a fine-print
appearance?   _____   _____

Is there plenty of white space on each page with wide
margins and three spaces between sections?   _____   _____

Is your most relevant experience highlighted by centered
headlines, underlines, or other emphatic treatment?   _____   _____

Does it conform with the accepted (but not strict) rule
of one page for each ten years' experience or less,
two pages for more than ten?   _____   _____

ORGANIZATION

Is your name, address, and telephone number included on
the top of the first page?   _____   _____

	YES	**NO**
Is your name at the top of each page?	_____	_____
Have you omitted your business address unless compelling reasons exist for including it?	_____	_____
Have you included your business phone number only if it involves no risk to you?	_____	_____
Have you avoided writing your resume as a one-page synopsis plus a detailed account that runs to three pages or more?	_____	_____
Is your strongest qualifying experience described first, followed by the next strongest and so on?	_____	_____
Is your highest education shown first in the education section?	_____	_____

CONTENT

	YES	NO
Are marginal leads, underlined statements, or other attention getters stated in terms of your accomplishments?	_____	_____
Does the content, wherever possible, emphasize results produced, interesting problems solved, significant achievements, etc.?	_____	_____
Have you avoided a straight recitation of duties and responsibilities that fails to show how well you did your job?	_____	_____
Where possible, have you used very short quotations from others that reflect credit on your performance?	_____	_____
Does your experience description cover your whole career, even if very briefly, with regard to early or unrelated experience?	_____	_____
Have you deemphasized experience not related to the job in question (even if very strong) and experience that is more than ten years old?	_____	_____
Does your section on education cover all important aspects of your schooling that add merit to your application – honors, high class standing, activities, scholarships, etc.?	_____	_____
Have you given due emphasis to awards, accomplishments, or activities in school, your community or elsewhere that support your credentials?	_____	_____

	YES	NO

Are any pertinent publications, professional associations, licenses, etc., covered?   _____   _____

Have you avoided including frivolous or potentially contro- versial activities or associations?   _____   _____

Have you avoided indicating conflicts in previous employment or other negative factors?   _____   _____

Have you eliminated such data as your social security number, religion, race, age, marital, and health status?   _____   _____

Have you left out location preferences, pay, or pay requirements?   _____   _____

Have you eliminated mention of references?   _____   _____

Have you omitted the date your resume was prepared and your availability date?   _____   _____

Have you included every major significant factor that supports favorable consideration for the job you seek?   _____   _____

WRITING STYLE

Have you phrased your resume to prove your ability to perform successfully on the job you seek?   _____   _____

Have you used short, dynamic sentences?   _____   _____

Is the grammar and punctuation correct?   _____   _____

Do all statements appear in proper syntax?   _____   _____

Is the spelling correct?   _____   _____

Is all detail unnecessary to a broad appreciation of your abilities and assets eliminated?   _____   _____

Have you avoided long words, overly descriptive adjectives, and superlatives?   _____   _____

Are you comfortable with everything your resume says and sure that nothing is exaggerated?   _____   _____

Are all laudatory quotations extremely brief and in smooth reading context?   _____   _____

Have you avoided technical jargon?   _____   _____

	YES	**NO**

Do most of your sentences start with action words
such as: directed, supervised, developed, planned,
produced, achieved, etc.?   _____   _____

Is "I" used sparingly, if at all?   _____   _____

Have you avoided an unduly modest approach and let the
facts speak clearly for themselves?   _____   _____

Does your resume avoid general statements regarding
your performance instead of specific facts?   _____   _____

Where possible, do you cite specific examples of
successful performance?   _____   _____

Do such examples quantify results – e.g., "decreased
turnover by 25% among nurses on my staff?"   _____   _____

OVERVIEW

Is your resume an attractive, interesting, quick-reading,
factual account that proves that your experience and
personal assets qualify you for the job you want?   _____   _____